Table of Contents

PREVIEW

Osteoarthritis, also known as degenerative joint disease (DJD), is the most common type of arthritis. Osteoarthritis is more likely to develop as people age. The changes in osteoarthritis usually occur slowly over many years, though there are occasional exceptions. Inflammation and injury to the joint cause bony changes, deterioration of tendons and ligaments and a breakdown of cartilage, resulting in pain, swelling, and deformity of the joint.

There are two main types of osteoarthritis:

Primary: Most common, generalized, primarily affects the fingers, thumbs, spine, hips, knees, and the great (big) toes.

Secondary: Occurs with a pre-existing joint abnormality, including injury or trauma, such as repetitive or sports-related; inflammatory arthritis, such as rheumatoid, psoriatic, or gout; infectious arthritis; genetic joint disorders, such as Ehlers-Danlos (also known as hypermobility or "double-jointed; congenital joint disorders; or metabolic joint disorders.

OSTEOARTHRITIS DIET RECIPES

BREAKFAST

1. Tender and Crispy Whole Wheat Banana Bread Waffles

Prep Time: 30 Minutes

Cook Time: 15 Minutes

Servings: 3-4

Ingredients

Dry ingredients:

- ½ cup whole wheat flour
- ¼ cup all purpose flour
- ¼ cup corn starch
- 1 tsp. baking powder
- ¼ tsp. baking soda
- ½ tsp. salt
- 1-2 tsp. sugar, to taste

Wet ingredients:

- 1 cup whole milk + 1 tsp. white vinegar or lemon juice (or just use 1 cup buttermilk)
- 1 large egg
- 1 small overripe banana, mashed (you want ½ cup mashed banana -- if your banana is really big, you might not need all of it)
- 1 TBSP melted coconut oil or vegetable oil
- 1 tsp. vanilla extract

Optional toppings:

- Slices of banana, chopped pecans / walnuts / hazelnuts, chocolate chips, nutella, whatever your heart desires.... and of course maple syrup!

Instructions

1. In a bowl or large glass measuring cup, whisk together all the dry ingredients.
2. In a separate bowl, mash the banana and mix in all the wet ingredients.
3. Add the wet ingredients to the dry ingredients, and mix well to combine. Let the batter sit, without stirring, for 30 minutes. Take a shower, make some

tea, and get the waffle iron hot -- just don't skip letting the batter rest! The batter might seem too thin at first, but it will thicken up as it sits.

4. Make waffles according to your waffle iron's instructions. Note: I find with most home waffle irons, it helps to go an extra minute or two after the waffle iron says it's "ready" before removing the waffle if you want a nice, crispy exterior. This will vary depending on your particular machine, so play around with the amount of time it takes to get your waffles to the desired level of crispiness.)

5. Serve immediately with sliced bananas, chopped nuts, and maple syrup. These waffles are best eaten the moment they come off the iron, but if you're set on everyone sitting down to eat at the same time, you can help preserve the crispiness a little by putting cooked waffles directly on the rack in a 150 degree F oven until you're ready to serve.

6. There are plenty of ways to mix up this recipe. Here are some suggestions:

For regular waffles: just omit the banana, and increase the oil to ¼ cup. (I like to use 1 tsp. sugar if I'm using a banana, and 2 tsp. sugar if not -- but that's totally personal preference.)

To banana bread waffles or regular waffles, try adding a pinch of cinnamon and nutmeg, or other spices like chinese five spice or ginger.

Swap the banana for pumpkin puree and a dash of pumpkin pie spices.

Make regular waffles, but stir in a spoonful of cocoa powder to the dry ingredients, and top with chocolate chips. (For add-ins like nuts and chocolate, I prefer to use them as a topping rather than adding them directly to the batter, so I don't have to worry about them burning to the waffle iron.)

For quick and easy waffles, I like to make a mix out of the dry ingredients. Just whisk together 5 or 6 times the dry ingredients in a bowl, store in an airtight container, and when you want to make waffles, scoop 1 cup of mix and follow the recipe as written. You can also make smaller or larger batches of waffles easily, just be sure to adjust the wet ingredients accordingly (i.e., for half a cup of mix, halve the wet ingredients).

Prep Time: 5 Minutes

Cook Time: 45 Minutes

Servings: 8

Ingredients

- 3 cups rolled oats (or certified gluten-free oats)
- 6 Tbsp light brown sugar, plus 1 TBSP
- 2 tsp. Cinnamon (we like to use rounded tsp, but you can use more or less, to taste)
- ¼ tsp. ground ginger
- ⅛th cloves
- ½ tsp. fine grain sea salt
- 1½ cups milk (or dairy free substitute)
- 1½ cups unsweetened applesauce
- 4 TBSP butter, melted (or coconut oil)
- 2 tsp. pure vanilla extract (if gluten-free, be sure to use gluten-free extract)
- 2 small apples, cut into ½ inch cubes (about 2 cups)
- Optional: 1 cup walnuts, pecans, raisins, or other mix-ins
- 1-2 apples, thinly sliced, for garnishing the top

Instructions

1. Preheat oven to 350 degrees F.

2. In a large bowl, combine all of the ingredients except 1 TBSP brown sugar, and the sliced apples. Dump the mixture into a 9x13 inch baking dish. Arrange the sliced apples on top, and sprinkle with the remaining TBSP brown sugar.

3. Bake on the center rack for 45-50 minutes, or until the apples are crisp-tender.

4. Remove from the oven and let cool for ten minutes before serving. Serve as is, or with a drizzle of maple syrup or honey, OR make it dessert with a scoop of ice cream or a dollop of whipped cream.

5. Leftovers can be stored in an airtight container in the fridge for up to a week, and can be re-warmed in a toaster oven or microwave before serving.

6. Can be easily made vegan / gluten-free by swapping coconut oil for the butter, dairy-free milk for the cows milk, and gluten-free rolled oats. (If you're cooking for someone who is gluten intolerant or has a serious allergy, be sure to use gluten-free vanilla extract, too.)

I love to make this oatmeal on the weekends, and have breakfast (or dessert!) ready for the rest of the week.

If you'd prefer to make a smaller batch, you can easily halve the recipe and bake it in an 8x8 inch baking dish for 35-40 minutes, and it'll be just as great!

Prep Time: 10 Minutes

Cook Time25 Minutes

Serves: 16-18

Ingredients

Base:

- 12 large eggs
- ½ cup heavy cream
- ¼ cup milk
- 2 TBSP fresh parsley, chopped
- 2 TBSP fresh basil, chopped (or other herb)
- ¼ tsp. salt
- ¼ tsp. pepper

Veggies:

- 1 cup broccoli, cut into teeny tiny florets
- 1 cup fresh spinach, roughly chopped
- 1 red bell pepper, chopped small
- ¼-1/2 cup onion, diced fine
- 1 jalapeno pepper, seeds and veins removed, diced fine (optional)

Add-ins (optional):

- 1½ cups cheddar, gruyere, mozzarella, or other cheese, divided
- 1 lb. bacon, sausage, or other meat, fully cooked

Instructions

1. If using meat (bacon, sausage, etc.), cook it fully first. Set it aside to cool, then cut into small pieces.
2. Preheat oven to 375 degrees F., and thoroughly grease (butter, coconut oil, or non-stick spray) a muffin tin. (NOTE: I recommend using a non-stick muffin tin for even easier removal.)
3. In a large bowl, whisk together the eggs, cream, milk, parsley, basil, salt, and pepper. Set aside.
4. Get all your veggies diced up and ready to go. Optionally, you can saute your onion with a bit of olive oil to soften it up and take away some of its bite. Set aside and allow to cool.
5. Add all the veggies to the bowl with the egg mixture, and stir to combine. Stir in half of the cheese, and all of the meat, if using.
6. Using an ice-cream scoop or ¼ cup measure, scoop the mixture into the prepared muffin pan. Fill to

about ¼ inch from the top, then sprinkle a small amount of reserved cheese over each. Place in the oven, and bake for 20-25 minutes, or until the egg is fully set and the cheese has just started to turn golden on top.

7. Remove from the oven and let cool for 5-10 minutes before running a butterknife around each muffin, and gently removing from the pan. Enjoy while warm, or let cool completely before storing in an airtight container in the fridge. Leftovers can be reheated for several seconds in the microwave (time will vary depending on your microwave), or a few minutes in a preheated oven or toaster oven.

8. Feel free to sub in whatever veggies you like, or have on hand. I used about 3-4 cups of chopped veggies in total, and wouldn't suggest using much more, otherwise you won't have enough egg mixture to go 'round.

Prep Time: 10 Minutes

Cook Time: 35 Minutes

Serves: 1 loaf

Ingredients

- 1¾ cups (210 grams) all-purpose flour
- 1 tsp. Baking soda
- 1 tsp. Baking powder
- ¾ tsp. Kosher salt
- ¾ tsp. Cinnamon
- ½ tsp. powdered ginger (or 1 tsp. Freshly grated ginger)
- 2 large eggs
- ¼ cup coconut oil, melted, plus more for greasing the pan
- 1 cup granulated sugar
- 2 tsp. pure vanilla extract
- 1 tsp. fresh lemon juice
- 1 cup shredded zucchini
- 1 cup shredded carrot

- 1 cup grated apple (I used red, but you can use whatever variety you like)

Optional:

- 1 cup chopped nuts, minced candied ginger, dried fruit, or other add-ins

Instructions

1. Preheat oven to 325degrees F.. Grease a 8x4 inch baking dish (I used coconut oil, but you can use butter or a spray if you prefer), then line the bottom with parchment paper. Stash the pan in the fridge or freezer to chill while you make the batter.
2. In a bowl, whisk together the flour, baking soda, baking powder, salt, cinnamon, and ginger. Set aside.
3. In a separate bowl, whisk the eggs until light and frothy. Add the coconut oil, sugar, vanilla, and lemon juice, and beat well for one minute. Grate the zucchini, carrots, and apple on the large side of a box grater, and add them to the wet ingredients. Stir to combine.
4. Add the dry ingredients to the wet, and fold them in gently until just combined, with no dry patches. The

batter will be quite thick, but that's how it should be --
a lot of the moisture is contained in the veggies and
apple, and will come out during baking to keep the
loaf moist. Do not over-mix.

5. Pour the batter into the prepared pan, and bake for
    55-65 minutes, or until the top is golden brown and a
    toothpic inserted in the center comes out mostly
    clean.

6. Let cool for at least 15-20 minutes before removing
    from the pan, then let cool completely. Serve
    immediately, or wrap in plastic and store at room
    temperature. Keeps beautifully for 3-4 days.

7. (I haven't tried making this loaf with any other kinds
    of flour yet, but plan on experimenting with a gluten-
    free version soon. I'll update here when I do!)

Prep Time: 10 Minutes

Cook Time: 35 Minutes

Serves: 3

Ingredients

- 2½ cups fresh rhubarb, chopped into ½ inch pieces (about 10 oz.)
- 2½ cups fresh strawberries, hulled and quartered (about 11 oz.)
- 3 cups granulated sugar
- 2 Tbsp fresh lemon juice (about one lemon)
- 2 Tbsp powdered pectin

Instructions

1. Place a small plate or saucer in the freezer before you begin, so that you can test the jam towards the end of cooking.
2. (Optional) If you're planning on canning the jam, bring a large stock pot full of water to a boil, and cook your (clean and empty) jars and lids for several

minutes to sterilize them. Remove the jars carefully using canning tongs, and set on a clean dish towel to dry. Keep the stock pot of water at the ready for sealing the jars.

3. In a large pot (not aluminum, as it may react with the acids in the jam), combine the fruit, sugar, pectin, and half of the lemon juice. Place over medium heat, and cook until the strawberries have released their juices and the sugar has dissolved, stirring frequently to prevent the sugar from scorching.

4. Once the sugar has dissolved, increase heat to high and bring to a rolling boil, skimming away any foam that appears at the surface. Boil for 5-10 minutes, or until the fruit has started to break down, stirring occasionally. To test the jam, spoon a small amount onto the saucer that's been chilling in the freezer. This will give you an idea of how thick the jam will be once it's cooled. If the jam sets up to your liking, it is done. If it's too loose, cook a few minutes longer and test again.

5. Once the jam starts to set up to your liking, remove from the heat and stir in the remaining TBSP of lemon juice. If you prefer your jam to be less chunky, use the back of a spoon or a potato masher to crush the fruit.

6. Carefully spoon the hot jam into the clean jars (a canning funnel is a big help, if you have one) leaving about ½ inch of head room in each jar. Once the jars are filled, wipe the rims with a damp paper towel to ensure a clean seal, and screw on the lids (or, if you're using weck jars, clamp the lids in place carefully).

7. (Optional) if you want to preserve your jam, return the jars to the stock pot of boiling water, lowering them in carefully with canning tongs, and making sure the water is deep enough to cover the jars completely. Cover the pot with a lid and let the jars process in the water bath for about 6-8 minutes. Remove the jars and set them carefully onto a kitchen towel. Let sit at room temperature until completely cool. If using ball jars, the metal lids should make a "pop" or "ting" sound as they cool, and the bump in the center of the lid should not flex when pushed down on, letting you know the jars have properly sealed. If any jars don't seal completely, store these in the fridge and use within a few weeks. Jars that are properly sealed can be kept in a cool dark place for several months or more.

8. I find Three cups of sugar to be the perfect amount, and makes a sweet, but still very brightly flavored jam.

However, it is on the low side as far as jams go (many jams use more sugar than fruit). If you prefer your jam to be even sweeter, feel free to add more sugar according to your tastes. If you're not sure, start with three cups, then taste the jam when you let it cool on the saucer. If it isn't sweet enough, add more sugar to the pot, and let it dissolve completely before testing again.

The amount of pectin used in this recipe creates a jam that sets up slightly, but isn't as firm as store bought jams. If you prefer a firmer jam, you can increase the pectin by another TBSP. If you prefer a looser jam, or want to avoid using pectin, you can omit it all together and cook the jam longer until it reduces and thickens slightly. (The reason I use pectin is it reduces the cooking time (my jam started to set after about 5 minutes of boiling), whereas a jam made without pectin will need boil significantly longer. Cooking the jam longer will reduce the overall yield, and can dull the flavor. If you don't have any pectin, you can try quartering a green apple and adding it to the jam at the beginning of cooking. This will impart some natural pectin, and you can remove it before spooning the jam into jars.)

Prep Time: 25 Minutes

Cook Time: 45 Minutes

Serves: 10-15

Ingredients

- 1 1/2 cups whole milk
- 1/4 cup white vinegar
- 2 cups all-purpose flour
- 1/4 cup dark brown sugar, packed
- 2 tsp. baking powder
- 1 tsp. baking soda
- 1 tsp. sea salt
- 1 1/2 tsp. cinnamon
- 1 tsp. nutmeg
- 1/2 tsp. ground ginger
- pinch of cloves
- 2 large eggs
- 1 cup unsweetened pumpkin puree
- 4 Tbsp unsalted butter, melted

Optional:

- Chopped pecans, or walnuts, or chocolate chips, to taste
- Maple syrup, butter, whipped cream, etc., for serving
- Or substitute 1 TBSP pumpkin pie spice. If you prefer your pumpkin pancakes plain, go ahead and omit the spices all together.

Instructions

1. To keep finished pancakes warm until serving, pre-heat oven to 200f.
2. In a glass measuring cup or bowl, stir together the milk and vinegar. Set aside to sour while you prep your other ingredients.
3. In a large bowl, whisk together the flour, sugar, baking powder/soda, salt, and spices if using. Try to make sure there are no clumps of brown sugar.
4. In another bowl, combine the buttermilk, pumpkin puree, eggs, vanilla, and melted butter. Add the wet ingredients to the dry ingredients, and mix until just combined – the batter will be lumpy, but that's okay. Over-mixing will cause tougher, gummier pancakes.

5. Place your griddle or skillet over medium-low heat – if you're making the jack-o-lantern flapjacks, you don't want the batter to cook too quickly and burn while you're still making your design. If your using a non-stick surface, do not grease it. If you do oil your pan, use very little.

6. To make the jack-o-lantern faces, pour some of the pancake batter into a plastic squeeze bottle, or an empty (and thoroughly cleaned) ketchup bottle or the like. Onto the griddle or skillet, squeeze two triangles for eyes, and make a mouth; or, draw a spider-web or other design. Once the batter begins to look dry on top, pour or squeeze more batter over your masterpiece. Because your drawing was on the heat first, it will cook longer and turn darker than the rest of the pancake. If you're using nuts, chocolate chips, or other add-ins, sprinkle a small handful on top of the pancake just before flipping. Cook until bubble just barely begin breaking on the surface, and flip your flapjack to reveal your design! Let cook for another minute or so, or until the underside is lightly browned.

7. Troubleshooting: If the batter in your squeeze bottle is too thick, you can add another tsp or two of milk. If

lumps in the batter are clogging the nozzle, you may need to cut a wider opening at the tip. If you pipe your design, and then the image moves around on the pan when you pour more batter on top, your griddle has too much grease on it – wipe it off with a paper towel and try again. If you plan on piping words into your pancakes, remember to write them backwards on the pan, since the image will be mirrored once flipped.

8. It might take a pancake or two to get a feel for how long to leave the batter on the pan to get the right color on it, and you may need to adjust the heat depending on your stove top.

9. Place cooked pancakes onto a plate or tray, and place in the warm oven until ready to serve.

10. Serve with fresh whipped cream, maple syrup, or garnished with more nuts or chocolate chips. Enjoy!

7.   Roasted Pear and Gorgonzola Salad with Balsamic Vinaigrette

Prep Time: 30 Minutes

Cook Time: 55 Minutes

Serves: 4-6

Ingredients

For the dressing:

- 3 Tbsp good-quality balsamic vinegar
- 1 Tbsp maple syrup
- 1 tsp. dijon mustard
- 1/2-3/4 cup extra virgin olive oil
- pinch of salt, to taste

For the salad:

- 4 firm, not-quite ripe pears (I used bartlett, but use what you like)
- 1 Tbsp butter, melted (or coconut oil)
- 1 Tbsp dark brown sugar
- 3/4-1 cup walnuts, or pecans
- 8 cups or so of mixed salad greens (I used arugula, spinach, red leaf lettuce, and baby kale, but frisee,

radichio, chard, and escarole are all in season in the fall, too)

- 1/4-1/2 cup dried cranberries, or cherries
- 1/4-1/2 cup gorgonzola cheese, or other crumbly blue cheese

Instructions

For the dressing:

1. Whisk together all the ingredients except the olive oil and salt. While whisking, pour in the olive oil. Start with a half cup, and adjust to taste. Add a pinch of salt, to taste. Cover and place in the fridge until ready to use. Whisk well before using. (Dressing can be made up to a week in advance.)

For the salad:

2. Preheat the oven to 400 degrees F., and line a rimmed baking sheet with aluminum foil or parchment.
3. Cut the pears into wedges (I cut mine into 1/8ths), and remove the stems and cores. Toss with the melted butter and brown sugar, and spread onto prepared baking sheet. Roast for 10-12 minutes, or until just tender (not mushy).

4. Meanwhile, place the walnuts (or pecans) into a dry skillet over medium heat. Toast for 6-8 minutes, or until warm and flavorful. Give the pan a shake, or stir the nuts, every couple of minutes to keep them from burning — keep your eye on them!

5. Combine your mixed greens, dried cranberries (or cherries), and crumbled cheese. When you are ready to serve, add the toasted nuts and roasted pears, while still warm. (You can keep your pears in wedges, as I did, or cut them into bite-sized pieces for easier eating.) Toss with dressing, to taste, and serve immediately.

Prep Time: 30 Minutes

Cook Time: 45 Minutes

Serves: 4

Ingredients

- 2 cups cake flour
- 3/4 tsp. baking powder
- 1/2 tsp. kosher salt (or 1/4 tsp. table salt)
- 1/2 Cup (1 stick) plus 3 Tbsp unsalted butter, melted and cooled slightly
- 1/4 Cup heavy cream or whole milk, room temperature
- 3 Tbsp Meyer lemon zest (or regular lemon zest)
- 1 Tbsp fresh Meyer lemon juice (or regular lemon juice)
- 3 Tbsp chia seeds (or poppy seeds)
- 1 vanilla bean, seeds of (or 1/8th tsp. vanilla paste)
- 1/2 tsp. vanilla extract
- 4 large eggs, room temperature
- 1 1/4 cup granulated sugar

For the glaze:

- 1/4 cup Meyer lemon juice (or regular lemon juice)
- 1/4 cup granulated sugar

Instructions

1. Preheat oven to 350f. (180c.), and line your muffin or cupcake tins. (Alternatively, you can spray/grease a 9×5 inch loaf pan, as that's what the recipe was originally intended for).
2. Sift together the flour, baking powder, and salt – give it a stir to make sure everything is evenly combined, and set aside.
3. Melt the butter and let it stand for a minute or two, so that it's warm but not hot. Add the cream, lemon zest and juice, chia seeds, vanilla, and vanilla extract. Stir to combine. The mixture should be thick, like a pancake batter – if the butter begins to solidify, warm it in 10 second intervals in the microwave. Set aside.
4. Using a hand or stand mixer, beat together the sugar and eggs. You want the yolks to go from deep yellow to light, fluffy, and pale. After 4-5 minutes the mixture will seem like a heavy custard, and your beaters

should leave trails as they spin. Keep beating for another couple minutes.

5. Using a flexible rubber spatula, gently fold the flour mixture into the beaten eggs and sugar. Fold by swooping the spatula down through the center, and coming up the side of the bowl – be sure to scrape along the bottom. Once most of the flour is incorporated, add half, and then all, of the lemon/butter/cream mixture, folding in between additions. Fold just until everything is combined, being sure not to over-mix.

6. Evenly distribute the batter into your muffins or cupcake tins (or pour the entire batch into a greased 9×5 loaf pan). This should make approximately 20 regular-sized muffins, or 60-70 minis.

7. Place your muffins on the middle rack of the oven, and reduce the temperature to 325f. (160c.).

8. Bake for 20-22 minutes, rotating the pan half-way through to ensure even baking. For minis, bake for 16-18 minutes, or until golden on top and a cake tester or tooth-pic inserted in the center comes out clean. (Or, for a loaf, bake for about 1 hour and 10 minutes, or until the top begins to turn golden).

9. Return the oven temperature to 350f. (180c.) between batches.

10. Let the muffins rest for 1-2 minutes, then transfer them to a wire rack to finish cooling.

11. For the glaze:

12. In a small saucepan, bring the sugar and lemon juice to a simmer, stirring just until the sugar has dissolved. Remove from heat.

13. Brush the lemon syrup over the tops of the still warm muffins. After brushing all of them once, you should have plenty of syrup to go back and make a second, or even third, pass. Letting this soak into the cakes is key to the overall experience, so don't skimp!

14. Serve fresh and warm, or store in an airtight container at room temperature for up to a few days.

Prep Time: 10 Minutes

Cook Time: 30 Minutes

Serves: 1

Ingredients

- 1/2 cup rolled oats
- 1/2 cup water – or coconut milk, almond milk, or other
- 3-4 Tbsp unsweetened pumpkin puree
- 1/2 tsp. cinnamon, or to taste
- 1/8th tsp. nutmeg
- 1/8th tsp. ginger
- small pinch of cloves
- small pinch of salt
- 1/4 tsp. vanilla extract
- maple syrup or brown sugar, to taste
- dairy or non-dairy milk or cream, to taste
- chopped pecans, walnuts, or shredded coconut, to taste
- Use regular rolled oats, not instant

Instructions

1. In a microwave-safe bowl, add the oats and water. Swirl to combine, then microwave on high for 1 minute. Keep an eye on things, because as the water boils the oats rise up considerably, and may overflow the bowl. This will depend greatly on your microwave, and the size of the bowl you use. If you plan to microwave more than 1 serving at a time, use a fairly large bowl. If the oatmeal reaches the top of the bowl, stop the microwave for a few seconds before continuing.

2. After about 1 minute (time will vary depending on your microwave) remove the oats, stir in the pumpkin, spices, and salt, and return it to the microwave for another 30-40 seconds, or until the oats are tender. Stir in the vanilla extract, then top with maple syrup or brown sugar, dairy or non-dairy milk or cream, and nuts as desired.

Prep Time: 10 Minutes

Cook Time: 30 Minutes

Serves: 1

Ingredients

- 1/2 cup rolled oats
- 1/2 cup water – or coconut milk, almond milk, or other
- 3-4 TBSP pumpkin puree
- 1/2 tsp. cinnamon
- 1/8th tsp. nutmeg
- 1/8th tsp. ginger
- small pinch of cloves
- small pinch of salt
- maple syrup or brown sugar, to taste
- chopped pecans, walnuts, or shredded coconut, to taste
- whipped coconut cream, to taste
- To make whipped coconut cream, refrigerate a can of full-fat coconut milk overnight. In the morning, flip can upside down, open, and poor off the 'skim' milk.

Scoop out the fat left in the can and whip with a little sugar or spices to taste. I mixed in a little extra pumpkin puree to mine, but this is optional.

Instructions

1. In a small jar, or a bowl, combine all ingredients. Top with nuts if desired. I got all fancy and topped mine with coconut whipped cream and a dash of nutmeg, but I'll leave that one up to you. Put a lid on the jar, or place a small plate over your bowl, and refrigerate overnight. In the morning, viola! Instant breakfast.

LUNCH

Prep Time: 5 Minutes

Cook Time: 30 Minutes

Serves: 6

Ingredients

For the freekeh:

- 1 cup dry freekeh
- 2¼ cup water, or low sodium vegetable stock
- ½ tsp. fine grain sea salt
- For the rest of the salad:
- 2 big handfuls (maybe 4-5 cups) baby arugula, or mixed baby greens
- 2 ripe but still firm pears, thinly sliced or cut into bite-sized chunks (I used bartlett, but you can use any kind you like, or whatever is ripe)
- ½-3/4 cup toasted pine nuts (sliced almonds or roasted hazelnuts would also be amazing)

- Crumbled gorgonzola cheese, or goat cheese, to taste (totally optional -- leave it off to make this salad vegan)

For the dressing:

- 4 TBSP white balsamic vinaiger
- 4 TBSP extra virgin olive oil
- Pinch of salt and pepper, to taste

Instructions

2. Place the freekeh in a large, shallow skillet, and toast over medium-high heat for 3-4 minutes, stirring or shaking the pan every now and then. Add the water and salt, and increase heat to high. Once boiling, cover, reduce the heat to low, and set a timer for 20 minutes.

3. While the freekeh cooks, toast the pine nuts, slice the pears, and crumble the cheese (if using). Whisk together the balsamic vinaiger and olive oil, and add salt and pepper to taste.

4. When the timer goes off, the freekeh should have absorbed all the liquid and become tender, with just a bit of chew. If there's any liquid left in the pan,

remove the lid and cook for a minute or two longer until it has evaporated.

5. Allow the freekeh to cool for just a few minutes (it should be warm, but not hot), then dump it into a large bowl and add the pears, pine nuts, salad greens, and all of the dressing. Toss to combine, then top with crumbled cheese, or serve with the cheese on the side so people can add it to taste. Serve immediately.

6. I think this salad is best served warm, right after it's made. However, the leftovers are mighty fine, too. If you find you prefer it cold, the freekeh can be made in advance, chilled, and then mixed with the greens prior to serving.

To make this salad vegan, omit the cheese. To make it gluten-free, swap the freekeh for a gluten-free grain such as brown rice, millet, or quinoa. Just be sure to cook according to package directions, as they will each require different cook times and methods.

Prep Time: 1hrs 5 Minutes

Cook Time: 1hrs 30 Minutes

Serves: 6

Ingredients

For the turmeric rice:

- 1 cup short grain brown rice
- 2½ cups water
- 1 tsp. ground turmeric
- ¾ tsp. fine grain sea salt

For the peanut sauce:

- ½ cup creamy peanut butter (look for one with no sugar added, if you can)
- ¾ cup light coconut milk
- 1½ TBSP fresh lime juice (about half a lime)
- 1 TBSP soy sauce
- 1 tsp. crushed red pepper flakes
- ⅛th tsp. garlic powder

For the collard rolls:

- 1 bunch of collard leaves (about 8-10 leaves)
- 1 red bell pepper, cut into thin strips
- 1 english cucumber, cut into thin strips
- 2 large carrots, cut into matchsticks
- 1 or 2 avocados, cut into slices
- handful of sprouts
- ½-1 cup thinly sliced purple cabbage

Optional:

- some fresh cilantro, or other herb you like
- Turmeric rice, and peanut sauce

Instructions

For the turmeric rice:

1. Rinse the rice, then place it in a medium saucepan along with the water, turmeric, and salt. Set over high heat, bring to a boil, then cover and reduce the heat to low. Let cook, covered, for about 40 minutes, or until the rice is tender and the water has been absorbed. If the rice is still a little wet when it's finished cooking, remove the lid and let the water evaporate, over low

heat, for a minute or two. Do not stir, or the rice will become gluey.

2. Let cool slightly before filling your rolls. Rice can be made in advance. Once cooled, it can be stored in an airtight container in the fridge for up to a week, or portioned into freezer bags and frozen indefinitely.

For the peanut sauce:

1. Mix everything together in a small bowl. If the peanut butter is particularly dry or hard (as natural peanut butters can be if stored in the fridge) microwave for a few seconds to soften, or place in a small saucepan to warm.

For the collard rolls:

2. Get all your veggies and other ingredients (rice, sauce) ready before you begin.
3. Fill a large, shallow skillet (12 or 14 inches) with water, and bring to a simmer. While the water is heating up, fill a large bowl with cool water and add a handful of ice.
4. Wash the collard greens if they are dirty, then dunk one into the boiling water. I like to use the stem as a handle, and just shimmy the leaf back and forth a little to get it submerged. Let the leaf blanch for 20-30

seconds -- it will turn bright green, and soften up so it's easier to roll, and tender enough to eat. Remove from the skillet and plunge the leaf into the bowl of ice water. Repeat with the remaining leaves.

5. When you're ready to roll, pull a leaf out of the bowl and blot it lightly on a clean towel. Spread the leaf onto your counter or cutting board, stem-side-up (the stem forms a large ridge down the back of the leaf). Using a sharp, non-serrated knife, fillet as much of the stem off as you can without cutting through the leaf itself. By this I mean, hold your knife perpendicular to the leaf, and gently slice away as much of the ridge of stem as you can. This will make the leaf more pleasant to eat, and much easier to roll. Slice off the entire stem at the base of the leaf, and flip the leaf over.

6. Add a small amount of each ingredient in a line across the width of the roll, leaving enough room on the sides so you can fold in the sides of the leaf like a burrito. Once all my rice and veggies have been added, I like to add a spoonful of the peanut sauce, too.

7. To roll, fold the bottom of the leaf up over the ingredients, then fold in the sides. Use your fingers to hold the ingredients tight, and roll away from you until the roll is almost closed. You can finish rolling as

is, but I like to add a small dab more peanut sauce to the last little bit of leaf, so that it stick and holds itself shut a little better.

8. Slice the roll in half, and you're done! Repeat with the remaining leaves.

9. Serve with the remaining peanut sauce on the side, for dipping. I like to eat these while the rice is still slightly warm, but they also last really well in an airtight container in the fridge. I've kept them for up to a five days. If the peanut sauce becomes too thick after refrigeration, add a splash of water or coconut milk to thin it out again.

10. Turmeric   Rice   Notes: Turmeric has a (well earned) reputation for staining anything it touches yellow. Because of this, I recommend cooking the rice in a stainless steel or nonstick-coated pot on the stove, as opposed to an enamel-coated pot or a rice cooker, which may get stained. If you don't care about the color of your rice cooker insert, you can certainly try making your rice in there. For storing leftover rice, you can use plastic baggies, or glass pyrex containers, which I've found won't hold on to the color at all. In the event that a container or a wooden spoon get stained, you can fill a

pot with water, add a splash of bleach, and let things soak for an hour or two before washing with warm soapy   water. Cooking the rice is the most time consuming part of making these rolls. You can start the rice cooking, set a timer, and prep your other ingredients while it cooks, or you can make the rice in advance. I like to make it in advance and portion it into little sandwich baggies in the freezer. This way I can easily take out and thaw single portions for using in rolls like these, or serving with soup or other dishes. While the color is vibrant, the turmeric is by no means overpowering, so this rice goes great with other dishes, too.

Prep Time: 15 Minutes

Cook Time: 20 Minutes

Serves: 3

Ingredients

- 2 lbs cooked chicken, chopped or shredded (you can use white or dark meat, whichever you prefer, cooked however you like: pan-seared, roasted, grilled, or poached... my favorites are grilled thighs, or breast meat when I roasted a whole bird. I've also been known to grab a store bought rotisserie chicken when I'm in a rush -- they work just as well for this recipe, and are a great way to save time)
- 1 red apple, cored and diced (I like to use a sweet eating variety, like fuji or honeycrisp)
- 2 stalks celery, diced
- 1 bulb fennel, cored and diced
- 3-4 TBSP fennel fronds, chopped
- ½-3/4 cup dried cherries, roughly chopped (or you can use dried cranberries)

- ¾-1 cup real mayonnaise, to taste (depending on how creamy you like it -- I find that white meat needs a bit more, while dark meat is good with less)
- Salt and pepper, to taste
- Optional: ½-3/4 cup walnuts or pecan, roughly chopped

Instructions

1. Gently mix everything except the mayonnaise, salt, and pepper in a large bowl. Add about ½-3/4 cup mayonnaise, and mix to combine. Add more mayonnaise as needed to coat everything evenly. Taste, and add salt and pepper as needed.
2. Refrigerate for 1-2 hours before serving. Salad stores well in an airtight container in the fridge for up to a week.
3. This salad is delicious on its own, over a bed of lettuce, or as a sandwich or wrap. Soft sandwich bread is great, and brings back memories of my childhood, but I'm also a big fan of rustic french or italian bread. Just add some greens, a few slices of red onion if you like, and you're good to go!

4. I love to make a big batch of this chicken salad and
    keep it in the fridge for quick, healthy lunches
    throughout the week. Even for just the two of us, a full
    recipe never seems like too much. It's also great for
    taking to a potluck or sharing with friends. If you'd
    prefer to make a smaller batch, though, simply halve
    all the ingredients.

Prep Time: 10 Minutes

Cook Time: 20 Minutes

Serves: 3 Servings

Ingredients

The Basics:

- 6 large portabella mushrooms
- about ½ cup marinara sauce (storebought or homeade. This is simply tomatoes, garlic, salt, pepper, and olive oil cooked until thick and saucy.)
- 2-3 oz. shredded mozarella cheese (or other good melting cheese, or your favorite vegan substitute)
- Meats: pepperoni, crumbled sausage or bacon (cooked first), diced ham, shredded chicken
- Veggies: finely chopped green bell pepper, red onion, black olives, chopped artichoke hearts, mini button mushrooms (mushroom on mushroom action!), baby arugula or spinach, etc..
- Other add-on ideas: crushed red pepper flakes, finely chopped fresh basil (optional but recommended), tiny

pinch of garlic powder or cajun seasoning, a sprinkling of parmesan cheese, ranch powder, etc..

Instructions

1. Preheat oven to 450 degrees F., and (optionally, for easier clean-up) line a rimmed baking sheet with foil or parchment. Prepare all your toppings and have them at the ready (if you're using meats, cook them and set aside. Chop all your veggies, grate the cheese, etc.)

2. Wipe the surface of the mushrooms clean with a damp cloth, then remove the stems with a paring knife and scrape away the gills using a spoon. The gills are perfectly edible, but removing them will give you more room for stuffing, and help reduce the amount of moisture in the mushrooms.

3. Place the mushroom caps open-side up on the baking sheet, and roast for 12 minutes. Remove from the oven, and gently use a pair of tongs to pick up each mushroom and drain off any moisture that has pooled in it.

4. Return the mushrooms to the baking sheet, and add a small spoonful of marinara sauce to each. Top with a

little cheese, and then a small amount of whatever toppings you like. I made some with meat and some without. My favorite was the sausage / green pepper / red onion pizza. (Go figure, these were my dad's favorite pizza toppings, too.)

5. Once the pies are topped, return them to the oven. Let cook for about 5 minutes, or until the cheese is bubbly and golden. If you want, you can switch on the broiler in the last minute or two to get the cheese nice and browned. Once baked, you can add fresh ingredients like baby arugula or chopped fresh basil. Serve.

6. You can fill these porta-pizzas with anything you like. I've included some suggestions in the recipe above, but feel free to think outside the box and use what sounds good to you!

Prep Time: 10 Minutes

Cook Time: 10 Minutes

Serves: 2 Servings

Ingredients

For the sauce:

- 1 Tbsp tamarind paste
- 2 Tbsp water
- 2 tsp soy sauce (or gluten-free tamari)
- 2 Tbsp palm sugar, coconut sugar, or brown sugar
- ¼-1/2 tsp. Ground thai chilis, or cayenne pepper, or red chili flakes, to taste (or you can use fresh thai chiles, aka birds-eye chiles, for some real kick)

For the veggies:

- 2-3 TBSP coconut or peanut oil, divided
- 1 large egg, lightly beaten (if you want to make this dish vegan, you can swap the egg for tofu)
- 2 large or 3 small sweet potatoes, peeled and spiralized (about 2 lbs, or 8 cups once spiralized)
- 2 cloves garlic, minced

- 2 Tbsp water
- 1 red bell pepper, thinly sliced
- 1 cup bean sprouts
- 3 green onions, chopped (green and white parts), plus more for garnish
- ¼-1/2 cup fresh cilantro, chopped, plus more for garnish
- 1 cup roasted and salted peanuts, chopped, plus more for garnish
- lime wedges, for serving -- optional

Instructions

For the sauce:

1. Stir together all the ingredients in a small bowl, and set aside.

For the veggies:

2. Heat 1 TBSP oil over high heat in a large nonstick skillet or wok. (I typically use a 12 inch pan). Add the egg (or tofu) and scramble quickly. Remove and set aside.

3. Return the pan to high heat, and add the remaining 1-2 TBSP oil. Add the spiralized sweet potatoes, and

saute for 2-3 minutes, tossing with tongs. Add the garlic, give it a stir, and then add the 2 TBSP water. Cover immediately to trap the steam, and let cook for another 2-3 minutes. Remove the lid and check the noodles for doneness (you want them to be tender enough to eat, but not so soft that they're threatening to turn into mashed potatoes). If they're still a bit crunchy, cook for another 1-2 minutes with the lid off.

4. Add the sauce mixture to the pan along with the cooked egg, bell pepper, bean sprouts, chopped cilantro, green onions, and peanuts. Toss gently to combine.

5. Serve immediately with additional cilantro, green onions, and peanuts for garnish. (You can also add additional chili flakes, or sliced chilis, if you want some extra heat.) Optionally, serve with extra lime wedges for squeezing over.

6. To make this dish vegan, swap the egg for tofu. You can use soft tofu to mimic the scrambled egg, or firm tofu, cut into cubes. Whichever you like best.

To make it gluten-free, be sure to use a gluten-free tamari in place of the soy sauce.

Prep Time: 10 Minutes

Cook Time: 10 Minutes

Serves: 2 Servings

Ingredients

- 2 large sweet potatoes (about 2 lbs.), cut into 1/2 inch cubes
- 15 oz. black beans, drained
- 1 cup sweet corn
- 1/2 onion, finely chopped
- 3/4 cup quinoa, cooked
- 1/2 cup rolled oats (or almonds)
- 2-3 cloves garlic, minced
- 1 TBSP cumin
- 1 tsp. chili powder
- 1/2 tsp. coriander
- 1/2 tsp. paprika
- 1/2 tsp. oregano
- 1/2 tsp. salt
- 1/4-1/2 tsp. crushed red pepper flakes, or cayenne (more or less to taste)

- 1/4 tsp. cracked black pepper
- Oil for pan frying.

For the chipotle/cilantro cream:

- 2 cups raw cashews, soaked in water (can be replaced with 1.5 cups vegan sour cream or mayonnaise)
- 2 chipotle peppers in adobo sauce
- 2 limes, juiced
- 2 cloves garlic
- 1/2 cup fresh cilantro, packed
- Pinch of salt

For the fries:

- 2 sweet potatoes
- 2 TBSP olive oil
- 1 tsp. cumin
- 1/2 tsp. salt
- 1/4 tsp. cayenne
- a few grinds black pepper
- (for those who are anti-sweet potato – blasphemy! – you could always replace them with regular spuds.)

Instructions

1. Cube your potatoes (leaving the skin on) and either oven roast (400f.), steam, or microwave in a large heat-safe bowl with a couple TBSP water until tender – I find the microwave to be a real time saver, and takes about 6-8 minutes. Stop to give them a stir every minute or two, until mashably soft.

2. Meanwhile, cook your quinoa. A 1/2 cup of dry will make enough for the burgers, but feel free to make extra. Add the quinoa to a small pot over medium heat, and let it toast for a minute or two. Add double the amount of water, bring to a simmer, and cover. Let cook 12-13 minutes, turn off the heat, and let it sit without removing the lid for another 5 minutes.

3. Meanwhile, meanwhile... Add your oats (or almonds) to the bowl of your food processor and pulse until it looks like very coarse flour. About 30-40 pulses.

4. In a large bowl, combine about 2/3rds of the beans, and 2/3rds of the sweet potato. Mash with a potato masher until slightly chunky and not quite smooth. Add in the rest of the beans, sweet potato and all of the seasonings. Give it another mash or two, keeping some of the texture.

5. Add all the other ingredients, and stir to combine.

6. Heat a skillet over medium-high, and add a drizzle of oil. Form about 1/2 cup of the mixture into a tight ball, then press it between your hands into a patty. Place patties in the hot skillet and cook 4-5 minutes per side. Remove to a plate in the oven to keep warm, and repeat with the rest of the mixture. Add oil and adjust the heat on the pan as needed.

7. For the chipotle/cilantro cream:

8. If you're using vegan sour cream or mayo, simply combine all ingredients in your food processor.

9. If not, drain the cashews and dump them to the food processor. Add the juice of both limes, and blend until smooth. Slowly add 3/4 – 1 cup water, until the cashews are about the consistency of a thick sour cream.

10. Add the peppers and garlic, blend until smooth, and then add the cilantro. Pulse a few times to combine, and season with a pinch of salt to taste.

11. For the fries:

12. Preheat the oven to 400f.

13. Cut the sweet potatoes into thin, uniformly sized matchsticks. Toss with the oil, then the spices, and spread on an aluminum-foil covered baking sheet. Keep them spaced so they don't steam themselves.

14. Bake on the lower rack of the oven for 12-15 minutes, then take them out and stir/flip them over.

15. Return them to the oven, reduce the heat to 350f., and continue to bake for another 12-15 minutes.

16. Turn off the heat, and crack the oven door open. Let them sit in the heat of the oven to lose some of their steam for another 5-10 minutes before serving.

Prep Time: 1hrs 10 Minutes

Cook Time: 30 Minutes

Serves: 4-5 Servings

Ingredients

For the lentils:

- 1 cup (200g) green or brown lentils
- 2¼ cups water
- ½ tsp. fine-grain sea salt
- optional: 1-2 TBSP olive oil and/or lemon juice, to taste

For the pickled vegetables:

- 1½ - 2 cups thinly sliced vegetables -- red cabbage, turnips, red onions, beets, carrots, or any combination
- ½ cup white vinegar
- ½ cup water
- 1 TBSP kosher salt
- 3 TBSP sugar
- 8-10 whole peppercorns

- 8-10 whole coriander seeds

For the chicken:

- 1 lb. boneless skinless chicken breasts, cut into 1-inch thick strips or 1 inch cubes
- ¼ cup unsweetened greek yogurt
- 1 TBSP olive oiil
- 1½ tsp. ground coriander
- 1 tsp. ground cumin
- ½ tsp. ground turmeric
- ½ tsp. ground black pepper
- ¼ tsp. ground allspice
- ¼ tsp. ground cinnamon
- ¼ tsp. garlic powder
- 1 tsp. kosher salt (or ½ tsp. fine-grain sea salt)

For the garlic yogurt sauce:

- ½ cup unsweetened greek yogurt
- 3-4 cloves roasted garlic, or 1 clove raw garlic
- 2-3 TBSP finely chopped english cucumber
- 2-3 TBSP finely chopped fresh mint
- 2-3 TBSP lemon juice, to taste
- salt and pepper, to taste

- optional: ½ tsp. ground sumac, plus more for garnish (this is a common ingredient in middle eastern cuisine and has a lemony brightness in flavor. You can find it at most spice shops.)

Instructions

For the lentils:

1. Rinse the lentils and pick over them to make sure there aren't any stones. Place the lentils in a medium saucepan, add the water and salt, and set over high heat. Bring to a boil, then reduce the heat to maintain a barely-there simmer.

2. Cook for about 30 minutes, or until the lentils are tender enough to your liking. If there is still some water left in the pot when they've finished, you can drain them in a strainer. If they run out of water and aren't tender yet, add a splash more.

3. When finished cooking, taste, and add more salt if needed. Serve as is, or with a drizzle of olive oil and squeeze of lemon.

4. Lentils can be made in advance and stored in the fridge for up to five days.

For the pickled vegetables:

1. Place all the vegetables into a pint sized jar or other lidded container. Combine the remaining ingredients in a small saucepan, and bring to a simmer to dissolve the sugar and salt. Pour over the vegetables, allow to cool, then refrigerate for at least 8 hours or overnight. (I suggest doing this all in one jar. However, if you are using a vegetable like beets or red cabbage and don't want the other veggies to be stained pink, you can separate them into their own jars. If you do, you may need to double the amount of brine (water, vinegar, salt, etc.) to fill all the jars. I did it this way because I didn't want everything stained pink in the photos, but normally I wouldn't bother.)

For the chicken:

2. Whisk together all of the ingredients in a big bowl or gallon sized baggie, add the chicken, and mix until all the chicken is evenly coated. Allow to sit at room temperature for 1-2 hours, or in the fridge overnight.

3. To cook the chicken on the grill: preheat the grill so it's nice and hot, clean the grates and brush with oil. Skewer the chicken, place on the heated grill, and cook for about 3-5 minutes per side depending on the

heat of the grill, and how thick your chicken is. Grill until the pieces are cooked all the way through, then remove to a plate or cutting board and let rest for 5-10 minutes before serving. (Bonus tip, I prefer these metal skewers to wooden ones.)

4. To cook the chicken on the stove: heat an extra 1-2 TBSP oil in a large skillet over medium-high heat (cast iron is preferred to get a nice char, but a nonstick skillet will work too). Add the chicken and let cook for 4-5 minutes per side, or until cooked all the way through. Remove from the pan and allow to rest for 5-10 minutes before serving.

5. For the garlic yogurt sauce:

6. Mash the garlic into a paste. If you're using roasted garlic, this is really easy. If you're using raw garlic, you can grate it on a microplane like this one , or grind it in a mortar and pestle to get a fine paste.

7. Add the garlic to the yogurt along with all the other ingredients, and mix well. Taste, and add salt and pepper as needed.

To serve:

1. Add a little of everything to a bowl, and dig in!

2. If you're a garlic lover, you know that most middle eastern restaurants serve an amazing, thick garlic

sauce -- almost a paste, really -- with their shawarma. This garlic yogurt sauce is NOT that sauce. I took some liberties here and made something closer to a Greek tzatziki sauce (yogurt and cucumber). I love how the bright tangy flavor of the yogurt and clean taste of the cucumber and mint lighten up the flavors of this dish. If you'd rather try your hand at making a more traditional Lebonese garlic sauce, this recipe looks like a good one: For this garlic yogurt sauce, I strongly recommend using roasted garlic if you can. Roasting garlic is a simple way to mellow the flavor and take away the bite. This way you get a ton of garlic flavor without the overpowering, almost spicy quality that raw garlic can have. You can find my tutorial on how to roast a whole head of garlic here. The same principle goes for roasting cloves of garlic, too -- just peel as many cloves as you want to use, and continue with the tutorial from there. Shawarma recipe adapted from this . I love using yogurt for marinating chicken because the lactic acid tenderizes the meat and keeps it nice and juicy, plus it creates a wonderful char on the grill.

Prep Time: 20 Minutes

Cook Time: 5 Minutes

Serves: 10 Servings

Ingredients

- 1 lb. Brussls sprouts, trimmed and thinly sliced
- 2 cups red or green cabbage, thinly sliced (about ½ a small head, or ¼ large)
- 2 cups kale, thinly sliced (about 2-3 leaves)
- 1½ - 2 cups tart cherries, chopped (fresh, or canned and drained, or frozen and thawed and drained)
- 1½ - 2 cups walnuts, roughly chopped
- 1 cup dried cranberries, or dried cherries, roughly chopped

For the dressing:

- ¼ cup apple cider vinegar
- 2 Tbsp honey (or sugar, or other sweetener, to make it vegan)
- 1 Tbsp whole grain mustard
- ½ cup olive oil

- salt and pepper, to taste

Instructions

1. Trim the stem ends of the brussels sprouts, and discard any rough looking outer-leaves. Stand them up on the flat (cut) stem end, and carefully slice as thin as you can easily manage. (Or, if you have a slicer attachment on your food processor, you can use that.)
2. Thinly slice or shred the cabbage and kale, and chop the remaining ingredients. (If your cherries are canned or frozen, be sure to drain them thoroughly.) Add everything to a large bowl.
3. In a separate bowl or glass measuring cup, whisk together all of the dressing ingredients. Add a pinch of salt and pepper, to taste. If the dressing is too tart for you liking, add a bit more olive oil, and if it's not tart enough, add a splash more vinegar. Same goes for the honey and mustard -- adjust to taste, if you wish.
4. Pour dressing over the slaw and toss well (I find tongs are great for this) until everything is evenly coated. Can be served immediately, or covered with plastic wrap and stored in the fridge. Slaw will keep well in the fridge for several days.

5. If you have a choice between large brussels sprouts and smaller ones, I recommend going with the smaller ones, as they tend to be a little more tender and have a milder flavor.

I love this slaw with both dried cranberries and fresh tart cherries, but you could easily swap the cranberries for dried cherries, and leave out the fresh ones if you wish. I also think it would be fun to try with some fresh cranberries, thinly sliced, in place of the cherries when they are in season. Obviously, feel free to play with this recipe to your tastes. And if you come up with a great variation, tell me about it! makes a lot of slaw as written perfect for a party or a big family, or, you know but you can easily halve all the ingredients if you want less. (leftovers of this slaw are amazing piled high on a turkey sandwich, with a little smear of dijon mustard on the bread. So, maybe you don't want to halve the recipe after all!)

Prep Time:20 Minutes

Cook Time: 5 Minutes

Serves: 4 Servings

Ingredients

- 2 english or hothouse cucumbers, chilled
- 2 large carrots
- 1 tsp. salt
- 2 TBSP rice vinegar
- 1 TBSP fresh lime juice (about half a lime)
- 2-3 TBSP honey, to taste
- 1 tsp. Toasted sesame oil
- pinch of red pepper flakes, to taste
- ½-1 TBSP toasted sesame seeds
- 1 scallion, sliced
- 2 Tbsp fresh cilantro, chopped (optional)

Instructions

1. If you have a spiralizer, use it to cut the cucumbers and carrots into long noodles. (My carrots weren't big

enough to fit in my spiralizer, so I used a jullienne peeler instead -- if you don't have a spiralizer, a tool like this will do in a pinch, or you can slice the carrots and cucumber thinly with a knife.)

2. Place the spiralized cucumber into a strainer and toss with 1 tsp. kosher salt. Let the cucumber drain for 15-20 minutes to remove excess water.

3. Meanwhile, in a small bowl or glass measuring cup, whisk together the vinegar, lime juice, honey, sesame oil, red pepper flakes, and sesame seeds.

4. Once the cucumber has drained for a bit, spread it onto a layer of paper towels, or a clean dish towel, and gently pat out as much moisture as you can. Place the "noodles" into a large bowl, and add 2-3 TBSP dressing, to coat. Toss to combine, then garnish with additional sesame seeds, sliced scallions, and fresh cilantro. Serve immediately. (Leftover salad can be stored in an airitight container in the fridge for up to a day, but keep in mind that the cucumber will continue to release excess water as it sits. If your salad becomes soupy, you can drain the water from the bottom of the bowl before eating.)

Prep Time: 10 Minutes

Cook Time: 10 Minutes

Serves: 6-4 Servings

Ingredients

For the pita chips:

- 1-4 TBSP light olive oil, or refined (unflavored) coconut oil
- 1 large pita bread, regular or whole wheat (or 2-3 smaller ones)
- pinch of salt, to taste
- For the dressing:
- ⅓rd-1/2 cup fresh lemon juice, to taste (about 1½ - 2 lemons)
- ½ cup olive oil
- 1-2 cloves garlic, grated on a microplane or very finely minced
- 1 tsp. ground sumac
- ¾ tsp. kosher salt (or ½ tsp. table salt)
- ¼ tsp. black pepper

For the salad:

- 2 hearts of romaine lettuce, chopped
- 1 english cucumber, chopped into large bite-sized pieces
- 2 medium tomatoes (or a couple handfuls grape or cherry tomatoes) cut into large bite-sized pieces
- ½ cup flat leaf parsley, chopped
- ¼ cup fresh mint leaves, chopped

Optional add-ins:

- Thinly sliced radishes
- Thinly sliced red onions
- Crumbled feta cheese

Instructions

For the pita chips:

1. To bake the pita chips: drizzle pita bread with 1-2 TBSP olive oil or melted coconut oil, rubbing it to coat both sides, and sprinkle lightly with salt. Bake at 350 degrees for 8-10 minutes, or until golden and crispy, then let cool and break into bite sized pieces.

2. To fry the pita chips: cut or tear the pita bread into bite sized pieces. Heat 3-4 TBSP coconut oil (or other neutral, high-heat oil) in a skillet over medium heat. Add the pita, and cook, stirring frequently, until golden and crispy. Remove from the pan and toss lightly with salt.

For the dressing and salad:

1. In a glass measuring cup, whisk together all of the dressing ingredients. Taste, and adjust if necessary (if the dressing needs more acidity, add more lemon juice, etc., to taste).

2. Chop the romaine lettuce, cucumber, tomatoes, parsley, and mint, and place in a large bowl. (If you'd like to add radishes, red onions, or crumbled feta cheese, you can do so now.) Pour over enough dressing to coat, and toss to combine. Top with pita chips, and serve!

3. The pita chips can be baked or fried for this recipe, whichever you prefer. Baking the chips uses a bit less oil, and results in a lighter, more delicate chip. Pan frying uses a bit more oil, and gives you a sturdier, more robust chip that can hold up a little better to the dressing. I tend to bake them out of laziness, because I can toss the whole pita in the oven, set a timer, and

make the rest of the salad while it's cooking. The fried chips are tastier, but you have to keep a close eye on them to keep them from burning.

DINNERS

21. Simple Oven Roasted Chicken

Prep Time: 25 Minutes

Cook Time: 45 Minutes

Serves: 2-4 Servings

Ingredients

- 4-5 lb. roasting chicken, whole
- 2 Tbsp olive oil, vegetable oil, or butter
- 1-2 Tbsp salt
- 1/4-1/2 tsp. cracked black pepper
- Paprika or other herbs/spices – optional
- Onions, potatoes, carrots, lemons, etc. – optional

Instructions

1. Get your oven preheating to 450f.
2. Rinse the bird thoroughly under cool water, inside and out. If your chicken came with giblets, remove them and set them aside for making stock.

3. Pat the bird thoroughly dry with paper towels, inside and out. Try to get as much moisture off as possible. The dryer the bird, the crisper the skin will be. While the oven is preheating, let the bird rest at room temperature so it can warm up a little.

4. Pour your salt, pepper, and any other spices you choose into a small bowl (this way you can grab them later without contaminating everything with chicken-y hands). Get your oil ready as well, and cut up any onions, potatoes, etc. you'd like to use.

5. Give the chicken a final pat-down with a paper towel and place it in a baking dish or roasting pan breast-side up. Drizzle it front and back with oil, and rub it all around to make sure everything is evenly coated. Take a palm full of your seasoning mixture and rub it around the inside cavity, then rub the remaining seasoning mixture evenly over the outside of the bird. If you have any onions, potatoes, carrots, or other vegetables you'd like to roast, arrange them around the sides of the baking pan. You can also stuff a wedge of onion, lemon, or fresh herbs into the cavity of the bird for more flavor, if you like.

6. Place on the center rack of your pre-heated oven, and bake for 30 minutes. Reduce the oven temperature to

350f., and bake for an additional 20-30 minutes, or until the dark meat registers at least 170f. on a meat thermometer. Remove from the oven and let rest for 15-20 minutes before cutting in to.

7. For the chicken salad recipe below, cut or shred the chicken breasts (white meat) into a bowl and place in the fridge until chilled.

Prep Time: 20 Minutes

Cook Time: 30 Minutes

Serves: 6-8 Servings

Ingredients

- 1 lb. fusilli or other spiral-shaped pasta
- 1 pint cherry tomatoes, halved
- 8 oz. fresh mozzarella, either small balls or torn chunks
- ½ cup pine nuts, toasted
- 3-4 TBSP chiffonade of fresh basil, for garnish
- For the pesto:
- 1½ cups fresh basil, lightly packed
- ½ cup pine nuts, toasted (can sub walnuts or sunflower seeds)
- ½ cup freshly grated parmesan cheese (can sub pecorino)
- 5-6 cloves garlic, roasted (or 2-3 cloves raw)
- 2-3 TBSP fresh lemon juice, to taste
- ½-3/4 cup good quality olive oil
- big pinch of salt, to taste

Instructions

1. In a blender, combine all the pesto ingredients except the olive oil. While blending, drizzle in the olive oil until the pesto has reached desired consistency. Taste, and add more salt or lemon juice as needed. Set aside.

2. Cook pasta until al-dente, if serving the salad warm, or just past al-dente, if you plan to serve it cold or at room temperature. Reserve ¼-1/2 cup pasta water before draining.

3. Thin the pesto with 2-3 TBSP pasta water to create a more sauce like consistency, then pour the pesto over the pasta while it is still warm. Toss to combine, adding more pasta water as needed until the pasta is coated evenly.

4. If serving immediately, add the cherry tomatoes, mozzarella, and toasted pine nuts, and garnish with a chiffonade of fresh basil. If making in advance, cover and store in the fridge, then mix in the tomatoes, mozzarella, and pine nuts just before serving. If the pasta becomes too dry, add a little more pesto, or a drizzle of olive oil, as needed. Can be made up to a day in advance.

Prep Time: 20 Minutes

Cook Time: 30 Minutes

Serves: 6-8 Servings

Ingredients

For the dressing:

- 3 Tbsp fig preserves
- 1-2 Tbsp water, as needed
- 1 tsp. balsamic vinegar

For the salad:

- 4-5 slices bacon, cooked and roughly chopped
- ½ cup walnuts, toasted and roughly chopped
- 3-4 fresh figs (can be omitted if not in season)
- Crumbled blue cheese, to taste
- 4 oz. mixed salad greens (I particularly like arugula, or a mix with frisee or watercress, which all have a peppery bite to them and go well with the sweetness of the dressing, or you can use whatever you like)

Instructions

For the dressing:

1. In a microwave safe bowl, stir together the fig preserves and water. Microwave for ten second intervals to help loosen the fig preserves, and to warm the dressing through (it is best served warm). This can also be done in a small pot on the stove. Add the balsamic dressing, and adjust to taste (more fig jam can be added for sweetness, more balsamic for a bit more acidity, or more water if the dressing is too thick). Set aside.

For the salad:

2. Start by toasting the walnuts -- I like to do this in a dry skillet over medium-low heat. Keep a close eye on them, and stir or shake the pan every minute or so to prevent burning. They should be toasted and flavorful after about 5-6 minutes. Remove from the heat, and set aside.

3. Cook the bacon until crispy, then drain on a paper-towel lined plate. Chop, or roughly crumble.

4. While the bacon cooks, crumble the blue cheese, slice the figs, and get the greens in a bowl large enough for tossing.

5. Here's the most important part: when you're ready to serve, assemble the salad. Add the walnuts and bacon, while still warm, to the salad greens, along with the blue cheese and sliced figs. Pour the warm dressing over everything (dressing can be reheated in the microwave, or on the stove, if needed), and toss everything until evenly coated.

6. Divide into bowls, and serve immediately.

7. Yes, it matters that the salad be dressed like this. Something about every little piece being coated by a light, even layer of dressing brings all the flavors together. You could serve it up un-assembled, and have people assemble and dress their own bowls of salad, but I strongly recommend that they toss the salad well before digging in. What can I say, it really does make a difference.

Prep Time: 15 Minutes

Cook Time: 45 Minutes

Serves: 5 Servings

Ingredients

- Red and yellow bell pepper, thinly sliced
- Carrots, thinly sliced
- Cucumber, thinly sliced
- Avocado, thinly sliced
- Baby bella or shittake mushrooms, sliced thinly and lightly sauteed
- Bean sprouts, or other sprouts
- Cilantro – optional
- Thai basil – optional
- Rice paper / spring roll wrappers

Peanut Sauce

- 1/4 cup natural creamy peanut butter
- 1 clove garlic, finely minced
- 2 tsp. soy sauce, or gluten-free tamari
- 1-2 tsp. fresh lime juice

- 1/2 tsp. sriracha, to taste
- 3-5 Tbsp water or coconut milk, to taste
- Fresh chopped cilantro or green onions – optional
- to make vegan, replace the sriracha with cayenne powder, or crushed red pepper flakes, to taste

Instructions

1. In a bowl, stir together all of the peanut sauce ingredients, adding the water or coconut milk at the end to thin the sauce to desired consistency. Taste and adjust the flavors to your liking.
2. For the spring rolls, prep and slice all of the veggies and any other ingredients you plan to use for the filling Try to cut everything no longer than the length of a strip of bell pepper (a couple inches or so).
3. Fill a pie pan about a 1/4 inch deep with warm water, take one sheet of rice paper, and soak it in the water for 15-20 seconds, until pliable. Be careful not to soak too long, or it will tear too easily to handle. After one or two tries you'll get the hang of things.
4. Lay the soaked sheet of rice paper on a clean plate and begin laying out your ingredients near the end of the rice paper closest to you, right in the middle. Make a

neat little mound with the ingredients, then fold the left side of the sheet over the top of your filling, then the right. The two sides should meet, or almost meet, in the center of your filling.

5. Beginning at the end closest to you, start rolling the rice paper around your ingredients, using your fingers to make a tight bundle. For a quick and easy video tutorial on rolling spring rolls,

Prep Time: 15 Minutes

Cook Time: 40 Minutes

Serves: 6 Servings

Ingredients

- 2 Tbsp olive
- 2 Tbsp butter, divided
- 1 small shallot, minced
- 1/2 cup fresh shiitake mushrooms, chopped (or whatever mushrooms you like)
- 1 cup Arborio rice (or other risotto rice)
- 1/2 cup white wine (use what you like)
- 4 cups low-sodium chicken or vegetable stock
- 1/2 cup frozen peas, thawed
- 1/2 lb. fresh asparagus, blanched*
- 1/4-1/2 tsp. fresh lemon zest
- 1 TBSP fresh lemon juice
- 1/4 cup sun dried tomatoes, chopped
- 1/4 cup loosely packed fresh basil, chopped
- 1/4 cup freshly grated Parmesan or Pecorino cheese (plus more for garnish)

- Salt and fresh cracked black pepper, to taste

- .

Instructions

1. Place stock in a sauce-pan and bring to a simmer over medium heat.

2. In a separate pan over medium heat, add the olive oil, one TBSP butter, shallot, mushrooms, and a pinch of salt. Saute for 1-2 minutes, then add the rice and cook for another 4-5 minutes, stirring constantly.

3. Add the wine and continue to stir gently until almost all of the liquid has evaporated. This should happen pretty quickly.

4. Add one ladle full of stock to the rice mixture, and stir gently until almost all of the liquid has absorbed. This will take just a few minutes. Once most of the liquid is absorbed, add another ladle full of stock, and continue to stir. Repeat until most of the stock has been used, then give the rice a taste — it should be just a little chewy still.

5. When the rice is almost done, add in the peas, asparagus tips, lemon zest and juice, sun dried tomatoes, and basil.

6. Once the last ladle full of stock has been added and the rice is just barely al-dente, remove the pan from the heat and add one TBSP butter and the Parmesan cheese. Stir well until incorporated, then season to taste with salt and fresh cracked black pepper. If you prefer your risotto a little looser, add a bit more stock or water.

7. Top with shaved asparagus and serve immediately.

Prep Time: 28 Minutes

Cook Time: 55 Minutes

Serves: 4 Servings

Ingredients

- 2 dried New Mexican Chiles
- 2 dried Ancho chiles (sometimes called Pasilla chiles), or Guajillo chiles
- 2 TBSP olive oil
- 1/2 yellow onion, diced
- 4-5 cloves garlic, minced
- 1 1/2 tsp. ground cumin
- 1 tsp. chili powder
- 1 tsp. dried oregano
- 1 (10.75oz) can tomato puree (about 1 1/4 cups)
- Salt and pepper, to taste
- Optional: a dash of cayenne, or pinch of crushed red chili flakes, to taste

9. Place the dried chiles in a bowl or large glass measuring cup and pour enough boiling water over them to cover. Place a cup or small dish on top to keep the peppers submerged, if necessary. Let soak for 15-20 minutes.

10. Heat the oil in a saute pan over medium heat and add the onions. Cook for 3-5 minutes, or until the onions begin to soften. Add the garlic and cook for another 2-3 minutes, stirring occasionally to keep from burning. Add the cumin, chili powder, and oregano, and stir for 30-60 seconds to toast the spices.

11. Remove the dried chiles from the water, reserving 1 cup of the soaking liquid. Split the peppers in half with a knife and remove the stems and seeds — I find it helps to hold them under some running water to rinse all the seeds away. If you prefer a bit more heat, feel free to leave some of the seeds behind.

12. Add the chiles, along with 1 cup of reserved soaking liquid, to your blender or food processor. Add in the sauteed onion and garlic mixture and the tomato puree, and blend until smooth.

13. Return the pureed mixture to the saute pan, and cook over medium-low heat for 15-20 minutes, stirring

occasionally. If the sauce becomes too thick for your liking, add a little water to thin it down. Season to taste with salt and fresh cracked pepper, and adjust the level of heat with a a bit of cayenne or crushed red pepper flakes, if you want it spicier.

14. Sauce can be made up to a week in advanced, and stored in an airtight container in the fridge.

Prep Time: 28 Minutes

Cook Time: 55 Minutes

Serves: 4 Servings

Ingredients

- 4 large bell peppers
- 1 Tbsp olive oil
- 12 yellow onion, diced
- 3-4 cloves garlic, minced
- 1 jalapeno pepper, seeds removed, diced fine (or 1/2 poblano pepper)
- 2 tsp. ground cumin
- 1 tsp. sweet paprika
- 1/2 tsp. chili powder
- 2 cups low-sodium vegetable or chicken stock
- 1 cup quinoa, rinsed
- 1 roma tomato, diced
- 3/4 cup fresh or frozen sweet corn
- 1/2 cup black beans, cooked or canned, drained and rinsed
- 1/4-1/2 cup fresh cilantro, chopped

- 1 cup enchilada sauce
- Salt and pepper, to taste
- 1 cup cheese, shredded (I used cheddar, but pepper jack, mozzarella, or a mix would all work well)

For serving:

- More enchilada sauce, fresh chopped cilantro, sour cream, salsa, etc.
- The heat of the pepper is in the seeds and veins — if you want to kick the spice up a notch, leave some of the seeds and veins in. If you want it milder, a poblano pepper has a mellower flavor than a jalapeno.

Instructions

1. Preheat oven to 375f., and lightly grease a 9×5 baking dish. Cut the peppers in half lengthwise, remove the seeds, and place in the baking dish cut-side up.
2. Heat the oil in a large skillet over medium heat and add the onion, garlic, and jalapeno pepper. Saute for 5-7 minutes, or until softened, stirring frequently to keep the garlic from burning. Add the spices and cook, stirring, for 30-60 seconds more.

3. Add the broth and quinoa to the pan, stir, and increase the heat to high to bring to a boil. Once boiling, cover the pan and reduce the heat to low. Let simmer for about 15 minutes, or until the quinoa is tender and the liquid has been absorbed.

4. Once the quinoa is cooked, add the beans, corn, cilantro, and enchilada sauce. Stir to combine, then season to taste with salt and pepper.

5. Spoon the stuffing evenly amongst the peppers, and cover the baking dish with aluminum foil. Bake for 20 minutes, then remove the foil and top each pepper generously with shredded cheese. Return to the oven and bake for another 10-12 minutes, or until the cheese is melty and browned.

6. Serve with enchilada sauce, cilantro, and any other toppings you like.

Prep Time: 20 Minutes

Cook Time: 45 Minutes

Serves: 8 Servings

Ingredients

For the tarts:

- 1 box (2 sheets) frozen puff pastry, thawed according to package directions
- 1 1/4 to 1 1/2 pounds heirloom tomatoes, sliced 1/4-inch thick
- 1 pint cherry or grape tomatoes, sliced 1/4-inch thick
- 4 ounces good-quality goat cheese, roughly crumbled
- 2-3 tablespoons olive oil, for drizzling over
- sea salt and fresh ground black pepper, to taste
- 1 egg + 1 teaspoon water, for egg wash
- for post-oven topping:
- 4-5 large basil leaves, chiffonade
- good-quality balsamic vinegar, for drizzling

Instructions

1. Note: Fresh summer tomatoes are juicy; this we know. To help with making these tarts, I slice my tomatoes and place them on a plate lined with paper towels, which helps to catch any excess juice that could hinder the tart-making process.

2. Preheat oven to 400°F. Line 2 un-lipped sheet pans with parchment paper. Whisk together the egg and water until combined.

3. Place one sheet of thawed puff pastry on a lightly floured work surface. Using a rolling pin, gently press the dough to flatten and seal any fold marks (no need to make the sheet any larger; this is only to even out the dough sheet.) With a thin-bladed knife, slice the dough into fourths and transfer them to one of the prepared sheet pans, evenly spacing them on the sheet. Using the same knife, gently score the dough 1/2-inch in from the sides to make a border; do not cut the dough all the way through.

4. Cut your tomato slices to fit into the squares; because tomatoes are round and your edges are straight, take a circle of tomato slice and cut one side straight. Vary them (don't just cut them in half; see photos above) so you can make each one a little different. Use a few

slices of the cherry/grape tomatoes to fill in where the curves of the larger tomatoes have left gaps, staying within the scored lines on the pastry. Divide half of the goat cheese (1/2 ounce per tart) over top. Using a pastry brush, brush each square with egg wash. Drizzle a little olive oil over the tomatoes, and season with a little sea salt and fresh ground pepper. Repeat with the second sheet of puff pastry.

5. Bake in the lower third of your oven for 22-25 minutes, until the edges of the pastry are a deep golden brown and the goat cheese is tinged with a little bit of color at the tips. Serve immediately.

Prep Time: 10 Minutes

Cook Time: 35 Minutes

Serves: 4-5 Servings

Ingredients

- 2-3 cups cherry or grape tomatoes, halved
- olive oil, for drizzling
- 2 TBSP butter, divided
- 1 clove garlic, minced
- 5 cups water
- 1 tsp. fine sea salt
- 1 1/2 cups dry polenta (course cornmeal)
- 1 cup whole milk
- 1 cup sharp cheddar cheese, grated (or other good melting cheese)
- 1/2 cup fresh parmesan cheese, grated
- Salt and pepper, to taste
- Pesto, for serving

Instructions

For the oven-roasted tomatoes:

Preheat oven to 375f.

1. Halve the tomatoes, and place cut-side up on a baking sheet. Drizzle liberally with olive oil, and sprinkle evenly with salt. Feel free to add other seasonings, or fresh herbs like rosemary, if you like.

2. Bake on the center rack for 30-40 minutes, or until the tomatoes have begun to shrivel up at the edges. Remove from the oven and set aside.

3. For the polenta:

4. Place a pot of medium heat and melt 1 TBSP butter. Add the garlic and stir for one minute, or until fragrant.

5. Add the water, cover, and increase heat to high to bring to a boil. Once boiling, stream in the polenta and stir well. Add the milk, and reduce the heat to low.

6. Cook for 20-25 minutes, stirring frequently, until the polenta is thickened, and tender when chewed. Turn off the heat, dump in both of the cheeses, and add the second TBSP of butter. Stir until melted and combined.

7. Season to taste with salt and pepper. Serve with pesto and oven-roasted tomatoes.

8. Leftovers can be warmed up and served as-is, OR:

9. Lightly grease an 8×8 inch baking pan, and pour any extra polenta directly into it. This is best done when the polenta is still warm. Press the polenta into an even layer, let cool, and cover with plastic wrap. Chill in the fridge for a few hours or overnight.

10. Once chilled, the polenta will be firm enough to overturn onto a cutting board in one big slab. This can be sliced into squares or rectangles and baked or fried until golden and crispy. Delicious!

11. Enjoy!

Prep Time: 25 Minutes

Cook Time: 35 Minutes

Serves: 4 Servings

Ingredients

- 2 medium chicken breasts, cooked and shredded or cubed
- 1-2 stalks celery, chopped
- 1/2 large apple, chopped (red or green apple, use what you like)
- 3/4-1 cup toasted walnuts, roughly chopped (or pecans, or other nuts or seeds)
- 1 cup grapes, halved (or dried cranberries, cherries, or other fruit)
- 1/4 cup plain greek yogurt
- 1/4 cup mayonnaise
- 1 TBSP apple cider vinegar (or tarragon vinegar, or white wine vinegar)
- 1 TBSP fresh tarragon, chopped (or basil, oregano, rosemary, or other herb)
- Pinch of salt and pepper, to taste.

- I like to use a combination of mayo and yogurt to make this classic salad a little lighter. Feel free to use whatever you like.

Instructions

1. Shred or cube the chicken and place it in a bowl. Add the chopped celery, apple, and toasted walnuts.
2. In a separate bowl, stir together the yogurt, mayonnaise, vinegar, tarragon, and a pinch of salt and pepper, to taste. Add the dressing to the chicken mixture, and stir to combine.
3. Mix in the halved grapes last, to keep them from getting bruised. Taste and adjust seasoning if necessary. If the mixture is a little dry, add a bit more yogurt or mayonnaise.
4. Store in an airtight container in the fridge. Salad is best after a couple of hours, so the flavors have had a chance to mingle. Serve as is, in a wrap, on a sandwich, or however you like. You could even double the dressing and mix in some cooked penne for a pasta salad. I like mine simply with fresh lettuce and a bit of avocado. Enjoy!